ANGER MANAGEMENT FOR TEEN BOYS

An Emotional Mastery Guide for Boys On How To Control Anger and Gaining Self-Control

Alina Robertson

Disclaimer

information is therefore strictly at your own risk.

The views and opinions expressed in this book are those of the author and do not necessarily reflect the official policy or position of any organization or institution mentioned in the book.

Alina Robertson is not a licensed therapist, psychologist, or counselor, and the information provided in this book should not be considered a substitute for professional advice or treatment. Readers are encouraged to consult with qualified professionals for personalized guidance and support.

Table of Contents

Introduction

Jake sat slumped at his desk, fists clenched and jaw tight. He could feel the familiar surge of anger building inside him, like a volcano ready to erupt. It had been a rough day – first, a heated argument with his best friend over a misunderstanding, then a scolding from his teacher for forgetting to turn in his homework. Everything seemed to be going wrong, and Jake didn't know how to stop the mounting frustration.

As the bell rang, signaling the end of the school day, Jake stormed out of the classroom, barely acknowledging his classmates as he passed by. He could feel the heat radiating from his body, his heart pounding in his chest. All he wanted to do was escape – from the noise, from the pressure, from the overwhelming surge of emotions threatening to engulf him.

But as Jake stepped outside into the cool afternoon air, something caught his eye – a small bird perched on a nearby branch, its feathers ruffled by the gentle breeze. For a moment, Jake's anger seemed to melt away as he watched the bird, its delicate beauty a stark contrast to the turmoil raging inside him.

In that moment of stillness, Jake realized something profound – that anger, like the storm clouds gathering in the sky, would eventually pass. And just as the bird had weathered the storm, so too could he. With a deep breath, Jake made a conscious decision to let go of his anger, to release the tension that had been building inside him.

As he walked home, Jake couldn't help but feel a sense of relief wash over him. He knew that anger would always be a part of his life, but now he also knew that he had the power to control it. And with that knowledge came a newfound sense of freedom – the freedom to choose peace, even in the midst of chaos.

Adolescence is a time of tremendous growth and change, marked by a whirlwind of emotions, experiences, and challenges. For many teen boys, navigating this journey can feel like riding a rollercoaster, with highs of excitement and lows of frustration and anger. This book is designed to be your guide, offering practical strategies and insights to help you understand, manage, and ultimately harness the power of your anger.

Understanding Anger:
Anger is a natural and normal emotion that everyone experiences at some point in their lives. It's a response to feeling threatened, frustrated, or hurt, and it can manifest in various ways – from irritation and annoyance to full-blown rage. Understanding anger is the first step toward managing it effectively.

At its core, anger is often a signal that something is wrong or needs attention. It can be triggered by external events, such as conflicts with friends or family, academic pressure, or feeling misunderstood or unfairly treated. It can also stem from internal factors, such as low self-esteem, unmet expectations, or unresolved trauma.

Why Anger Matters for Teens:
Anger is particularly significant during the teenage years for several reasons. Firstly, adolescence is a period of intense emotional development, during which teens are learning to navigate their feelings and express themselves assertively. Anger, if left unchecked, can disrupt this process and lead to strained relationships, poor decision-making, and even violence.

Secondly, unresolved anger can have long-term consequences on mental and physical health. Chronic anger has been linked to a range of issues, including depression, anxiety, substance abuse, and cardiovascular problems. By learning how to manage their anger early on, teens can lay the foundation for a healthier and happier future.

Lastly, anger can be a powerful force for positive change when channeled constructively. It can motivate teens to advocate for themselves and others, stand up against injustice, and address underlying issues in their lives. By learning to harness their anger in productive ways, teens can become more resilient, empathetic, and empowered individuals.

Understanding what triggers your anger is essential for effective anger management. Triggers can vary widely from person to person, and they can be both internal and external. In this section, we'll delve into identifying personal triggers and recognizing external triggers, empowering you to better understand and manage your anger.

Identifying Personal Triggers

Personal triggers are those internal factors that can provoke feelings of anger. These triggers are often rooted in past experiences, beliefs, and values, and they can vary greatly from one individual to another. Identifying your personal triggers is the first step toward gaining control over your anger.

1. **Reflect on Past Experiences:** Take some time to reflect on past experiences that have led to feelings of anger. Was there a recurring theme or pattern? For example, you may find that you become angry when

you feel disrespected or when your boundaries are crossed.

2. **Explore Core Beliefs:** Our beliefs about ourselves, others, and the world around us can significantly influence how we interpret and respond to situations. Consider whether you hold any core beliefs that contribute to your anger. For instance, if you believe that you must always be in control or that you're not good enough, you may become angry when things don't go according to plan.

3. **Identify Triggers in Specific Situations:** Pay attention to situations or contexts where you tend to experience heightened levels of anger. Is it during conflicts with peers or authority figures? Is it in response to criticism or perceived injustices? By identifying common triggers, you can begin to develop strategies for managing them more effectively.

4. **Monitor Physical and Emotional Responses:** Notice how your body and mind

react when you encounter a trigger. Do you experience tension in your muscles, rapid heartbeat, or racing thoughts? Becoming aware of physical and emotional cues can help you recognize when you're being triggered and take proactive steps to de-escalate the situation.

5. **Keep a Trigger Journal:** Consider keeping a journal where you record instances of anger and the events or thoughts that preceded them. This can help you identify patterns over time and gain deeper insight into your personal triggers.

By taking the time to identify your personal triggers, you can gain greater control over your anger and develop more adaptive ways of responding to challenging situations.

Recognizing External Triggers

External triggers are factors in the environment that can evoke feelings of anger. These triggers can include specific people, places, situations, or events that elicit a strong emotional response. Learning to recognize and manage external triggers is crucial for maintaining emotional stability and preventing escalation.

1. **Identify Common Triggers:** Start by identifying common external triggers that provoke feelings of anger. This could include being criticized, feeling ignored or dismissed, or encountering situations that challenge your sense of fairness or justice.

2. **Pay Attention to Environmental Cues:** Notice how your surroundings impact your mood and behavior. Are there certain places or environments where you tend to feel more irritable or on edge? Pay attention to factors such as noise levels, crowding, or temperature, which can influence your emotional state.

3. **Recognize Triggering Situations:** Certain situations may inherently trigger anger, such as being stuck in traffic, waiting in long lines, or dealing with technology

malfunctions. By anticipating these triggers, you can prepare yourself mentally and emotionally to cope with them more effectively.

4. **Set Boundaries:** Establishing boundaries can help protect you from external triggers that are within your control. For example, if certain people consistently provoke feelings of anger, consider setting boundaries around your interactions with them or finding ways to limit your exposure.

5. **Practice Mindfulness:** Mindfulness techniques, such as deep breathing, meditation, or grounding exercises, can help you stay present and centered when faced with external triggers. By cultivating mindfulness, you can develop greater awareness of your reactions and choose more adaptive responses.

6. **Seek Support:** Don't hesitate to seek support from friends, family, or professionals if you're struggling to manage

external triggers on your own. Talking to someone you trust can provide perspective, validation, and practical advice for navigating challenging situations.

By recognizing external triggers and developing strategies for managing them, you can reduce the frequency and intensity of your anger, leading to greater emotional well-being and interpersonal harmony.

Understanding and managing anger triggers is a crucial aspect of anger management for teen boys. By identifying personal triggers and recognizing external triggers, you can gain greater control over your emotional responses and navigate the ups and downs of adolescence with greater east and resilience.

The Science Behind Anger

Understanding the science behind anger can provide valuable insights into how it affects the body and mind. From physiological changes to neural processes, anger is a complex emotion with a wide-ranging impact. In this section, we'll explore how anger affects the body and mind and delve into the neurobiology of anger.

How Anger Affects the Body and Mind
Anger triggers a cascade of physiological responses that prepare the body to react to perceived threats or challenges. When you experience anger, your body releases stress hormones such as adrenaline and cortisol, which increase heart rate, blood pressure, and respiration rate. This physiological arousal is often accompanied by muscle tension, heightened alertness, and a surge of energy, preparing you for fight or flight.

While these responses can be adaptive in certain situations, chronic or intense anger can take a toll on both physical and mental health. Prolonged exposure to stress hormones can weaken the immune system, disrupt sleep patterns, and contribute to cardiovascular problems such as high blood pressure and heart disease. Additionally, chronic anger has been linked to an increased risk of anxiety, depression, and other mental health disorders.

On a cognitive level, anger can impair judgment, decision-making, and impulse control. When you're angry, your brain's prefrontal cortex – responsible for rational thinking and self-regulation – may become less active, while regions associated with emotional processing and reactivity, such as the amygdala, may become more active. This imbalance can lead to impulsive or aggressive behavior, as well as difficulty in seeing situations from alternative perspectives.

Moreover, anger can impact interpersonal relationships, as it often leads to communication breakdowns, conflicts, and resentment. When individuals are unable to effectively manage their anger, it can strain relationships with family, friends, and peers, leading to feelings of isolation and loneliness.

Neurobiology of Anger

The neurobiology of anger involves complex interactions between various regions of the brain, neurotransmitters, and hormonal systems. At the core of the brain's anger circuitry is the amygdala, an almond-shaped structure located within the limbic system. The amygdala plays a central role in processing emotions, particularly fear, aggression, and anger.

When you perceive a threat or injustice, sensory information is relayed to the amygdala, which then sends signals to other brain regions, such as the hypothalamus and brainstem, to initiate the body's stress response. This triggers the release of stress hormones, which prepare the body for action and amplify emotional arousal.

In addition to the amygdala, other brain regions, such as the prefrontal cortex and anterior cingulate cortex, play important roles in regulating and modulating anger responses. The prefrontal cortex is involved in cognitive processes such as decision-making, impulse control, and emotion regulation, while the anterior cingulate cortex helps monitor and regulate emotional arousal.

Neurotransmitters such as dopamine, serotonin, and norepinephrine also play key roles in the experience and expression of anger. Imbalances in these neurotransmitter systems have been implicated in various psychiatric disorders characterized by dysregulated anger, such as depression, anxiety, and post-traumatic stress disorder (PTSD).

Understanding the neurobiology of anger can provide valuable insights into its underlying mechanisms and inform the development of more effective interventions for anger management. By targeting specific brain regions, neurotransmitter systems, and hormonal pathways, researchers and clinicians can develop tailored strategies for preventing and treating anger-related problems.

In conclusion, anger is a complex emotion with profound effects on both the body and mind. By understanding how anger affects the body's physiological responses and the brain's neural circuitry, we can gain greater insight into its underlying mechanisms and develop more effective strategies for managing anger and promoting emotional well-being.

Expressing Anger Constructively

Anger is a natural and valid emotion, but expressing it in a constructive manner is key to maintaining healthy relationships and resolving conflicts effectively. In this section, we'll explore two important aspects of expressing anger constructively: communication skills and assertiveness techniques.

Communication Skills

Effective communication is essential for expressing anger in a constructive way. It involves expressing your feelings clearly and assertively while also listening empathetically to the perspective of others. Here are some communication skills that can help you express anger constructively:

1. Use "I" Statements: When expressing anger, focus on your own feelings and experiences using "I" statements. For example, instead of saying, "You always make me angry," try saying, "I feel frustrated when..."

2. Be Specific and Concrete: Clearly articulate the behavior or action that is causing your anger, and provide specific examples if possible. Avoid generalizations or exaggerations, as they can undermine the validity of your message.

3. Stay Calm and Controlled: Maintain a calm and composed demeanor when expressing anger. Avoid yelling, name-calling, or using aggressive body language, as these can escalate conflicts and hinder effective communication.

4. Listen Actively: Be attentive and open-minded when listening to the perspective of others. Validate their feelings and show empathy, even if you disagree with their viewpoint. Active listening can help de-escalate conflicts and foster mutual understanding.

5. Seek Solutions: Focus on finding mutually acceptable solutions to the underlying issue rather than placing blame or seeking revenge. Collaborate with the other party to brainstorm potential solutions and work together toward resolution.

6. Take Breaks if Necessary: If emotions are running high and communication becomes hearted, it's okay to take a break and revisit the conversation later. Use this time to calm down, reflect on your feelings, and gather your thoughts before resuming the discussion.

Assertiveness Techniques

Assertiveness involves expressing your thoughts, feelings, and needs in a clear, respectful, and confident manner, while also respecting the rights and boundaries of others. Assertiveness techniques can help you assert your rights and communicate your anger effectively without resorting to aggression or passivity. Here are some assertiveness techniques to consider:

1. **Use "I" Statements:** As mentioned earlier, "I" statements can help you assert your feelings and needs without blaming or attacking others. For example, "I feel upset when you interrupt me during meetings. I would appreciate it if you could let me finish speaking."

2. **Set Boundaries:** Clearly define your boundaries and communicate them assertively to others. Assertive boundary-setting involves stating your limits firmly and respectfully, and being willing to enforce them if necessary. For example, "I'm not comfortable lending out my belongings without permission. Please ask me first before using them."

3. **Practice Active Listening:** Assertive communication involves not only expressing yourself but also listening actively to the needs and concerns of others. Show empathy and understanding, and demonstrate that you value their perspective.

4. Use Assertive Body Language: Pay attention to your body language when asserting yourself. Stand or sit up straight, make eye contact, and use a firm but calm tone of voice. Avoid crossing your arms, fidgeting, or avoiding contact, as these can signal defensiveness or insecurity.

5. Learn to Say No: Assertiveness means being able to say no when necessary without feeling guilty or apologizing excessively. Practice saying no assertively but respectfully, and offer alternatives or compromises when appropriate.

6. Use Assertive Conflict Resolution Techniques: When conflicts arise, assertive conflict resolution techniques can help you address the issue directly and assert your needs while also respecting the rights and feelings of others. Focus on finding win-win solutions that meet the needs of all parties involved.

By mastering communication skills and assertiveness techniques, you can express anger constructively, resolve conflicts effectively, and maintain healthy relationships with others. Remember that expressing anger constructively is not about suppressing or denying your emotions, but rather about expressing them in a way that respects both yourself and others.

Strategies for Managing Anger

Anger is a powerful emotion that, if left unchecked, can have negative consequences on our relationships, health, and overall well-being. Fortunately, there are several effective strategies for managing anger in healthy and constructive ways. In this section, we'll explore three key strategies: deep breathing and relaxation exercises, cognitive restructuring, and problem-solving techniques.

Deep Breathing and Relaxation Exercises
Deep breathing and relaxation exercises are powerful tools for calming the body and mind during moments of anger. These techniques work by activating the body's relaxation response, which counteracts the physiological arousal associated with anger. Here are some relaxation exercises you can try:

1. Deep Breathing: Practice deep breathing exercises to slow down your heart rate and promote feelings of calmness. Sit or lie down in a comfortable position, close your eyes, and take slow, deep breaths through your nose, filling your lungs with air. Hold your breath for a few seconds, then slowly through your mouth. Repeat this process several times until you feel more relaxed.

2. Progressive Muscle Relaxation (PMR): PMR involves tension and then releasing each muscle group in your body, one at a time, to promote relaxation and relaxation. Start with your toes and work your way up to your head, tensing each muscle group for a few seconds before releasing. Focus on the sensation of relaxation as you let go of tension in each muscle group.

3. Visualization: Close your eyes and imagine yourself in a peaceful, calming place, such as a beach, forest, or mountain retreat. Visualize the sights, sounds, and sensations of this tranquil environment, allowing yourself to immerse fully in the experience. Visualization can help distract your mind from anger-provoking thoughts and promote relaxation.

4. Mindfulness Meditation: Practice mindfulness meditation to cultivate present-moment awareness and non-judgmental acceptance of your thoughts and feelings. Focus on your breath, bodily sensations, or a specific object of meditation, and gently bring your attention back whenever your mind wanders. Mindfulness meditation can help you observe your anger without becoming overwhelmed by it.

By incorporating deep breathing and relaxation exercises into your daily routine, you can build resilience to anger triggers and cultivate a greater sense of calm and emotional balance.

Cognitive Restructuring

Cognitive restructuring involves identifying and challenging irrational or unhelpful thoughts that contribute to anger and replacing them with more balanced and rational ones. This technique is based on the premise that our thoughts influence our emotions and behaviors, so by changing our thinking patterns, we can change how we feel and react to situations. Here's how to practice cognitive restructuring:

1. Identify Anger-Provoking Thoughts: Pay attention to the thoughts and beliefs that accompany feelings of anger. Are there any recurring patterns or themes? Common cognitive distortions associated with anger include black-and-white thinking, catastrophizing, and personalization.

2. Challenge Irrational Thoughts: Once you've identified your anger-provoking thoughts, challenge them by asking yourself questions such as:

- What proof do you have to support this thought?
- Am I jumping to conclusions or exaggerating the situation?

- Are there alternative explanations or perspectives I haven't considered?

3. **Generate More Balanced Thoughts:** Replace irrational or unhelpful thoughts with more balanced and rational ones. For example, instead of thinking, "This is unfair and I can't stand it," try reframing it as, "This situation is challenging, but I can handle it. I'll focus on finding a solution."

4. **Practice Positive Self-Talk:** Use positive affirmations and self-encouragement to bolster your confidence and self-esteem. Remind yourself of your strengths, coping abilities, and past successes in managing anger. Positive self-talk can help counteract negative thinking patterns and build resilience to anger triggers.

5. **Seek Perspective:** Talk to trusted friends, family members, or a therapist about your anger-provoking thoughts and beliefs. Getting an outside perspective can help you challenge distorted thinking patterns and

gain insight into more constructive ways of interpreting situations.

By practicing cognitive restructuring, you can develop a more balanced and adaptive mindset that enables you to respond to anger triggers with greater clarity, perspective, and self-control.

Problem-Solving Techniques

Effective problem-solving skills are crucial for managing anger and resolving conflicts in constructive ways. Instead of reacting impulsively to anger-provoking situations, problem-solving techniques empower you to identify the underlying issues and work toward practical solutions. Here are some problem-solving techniques to try:

1. Define the Problem: Clearly identify the specific issue or conflict that is causing your anger. Break the problem down into smaller, manageable components, and consider the underlying factors contributing to the situation.

2. Generate Solutions: Brainstorm potential solutions to the problem, considering both short-term and long-term outcomes. Be creative and open-minded, and don't dismiss ideas prematurely. Even seemingly unconventional solutions may hold value.

3. Evaluate Solutions: Assess the potential benefits and drawbacks of each solution, weighing factors such as feasibility, effectiveness, and ethical considerations. Consider how each solution aligns with your values and goals, and prioritize those that offer the best overall outcome.

4. Make a Plan: Once you've selected a preferred solution, create a step-by-step plan for implementing it. Identify specific actions you need to take, resources you may require, and potential obstacles you may encounter along the way.

5. Take Action: Put your plan into action, and begin implementing the chosen solution.

Stay focused and committed to following through with your plan, and be prepared to adjust course if necessary based on feedback and new information.

6. Reflect and Learn: After implementing your chosen solution, take time to reflect on the outcomes and lessons learned from the experience. Celebrate successes and acknowledge areas for improvement, and use this feedback to inform future problem-solving efforts.

By practicing problem-solving techniques, you can address underlying issues, resolve conflicts, and prevent anger from escalating into destructive behavior. Effective problem-solving skills enable you to approach anger-provoking situations with a proactive and solution-oriented mindset, leading to more positive outcomes and healthier relationships.

Managing anger effectively requires a combination of strategies that address both the physiological and psychological aspects of anger. By incorporating deep breathing and relaxation exercises, cognitive restructuring, and problem-solving techniques into your anger management toolkit, you can develop greater emotional resilience, self-awareness, and interpersonal skills. Remember that managing anger is a skill that takes time and practice to master, but with dedication and perseverance, you can learn to navigate challenging situations with greater calm and confidence.

Developing Emotional Awareness

Emotional awareness is the ability to recognize, understand, and manage our own emotions as well as the emotions of others. It's a fundamental skill for effective communication, interpersonal relationships, and overall well-being. In this section, we'll explore two key aspects of developing emotional awareness: recognizing and naming emotions, and building empathy and understanding others.

Recognizing and Naming Emotions
The first step in developing emotional awareness is to recognize and name our own emotions. Many people struggle to identify and articulate their feelings, which can lead to difficulties in managing them effectively. Here are some strategies for recognizing and naming emotions:

1. Mindfulness Practice: Cultivate present-moment awareness through mindfulness meditation or mindfulness exercises. Pay attention to your thoughts, bodily sensations, and emotions without judgment, and practice labeling your feelings as they arise.

2. Check-In with Yourself: Take regular pauses throughout the day to check in with yourself and assess how you're feeling. Consider asking yourself inquiries like, "Which emotions am I currently feeling?" and "What factors could be influencing these emotions?"

3. Use a Feelings Wheel: Use a feelings wheel or emotion chart to help you identify and name specific emotions. These visual aids categorize emotions into primary and secondary categories, making it easier to pinpoint the exact emotion you're experiencing.

4. Journaling: Keep a journal where you can express and explore your thoughts and feelings in writing. Use descriptive language to articulate your emotions, and reflect on the underlying causes or triggers for each emotion.

5. Practice Emotional Vocabulary: Expand your emotional vocabulary by learning to differentiate between subtle variations of emotions. For example, instead of simply saying, "I feel bad," try to identify whether you're feeling disappointed, frustrated, or sad.

6. Pay Attention to Physical Cues: Emotions are often accompanied by physical sensations such as tightness in the chest, butterflies in the stomach, or a lump in the throat. Pay attention to these bodily cues as they can provide valuable clues about your emotional state.

By becoming more adept at recognizing and naming your own emotions, you can develop greater self-awareness and emotional intelligence, which are essential for managing emotions effectively.

Building Empathy and Understanding Others

Empathy is the ability to understand and share the feelings of others, and it plays a crucial role in building meaningful connections and fostering healthy relationships. Developing empathy involves stepping outside of your own perspective and tuning into the emotions and experiences of others. Here's how to cultivate empathy and understanding:

1. Practice Active Listening: When interacting with others, make a conscious effort to listen attentively and empathetically. Focus on understanding their perspective without interrupting or passing judgment. Reflect back what you hear to demonstrate that you're truly listening and understanding.

2. Put Yourself in Their Shoes: Imagine yourself in the person's position and consider how you would feel and react in their situation. This exercise can help you develop a greater sense of empathy and perspective-taking.

3. Ask Open-Ended Questions: Encourage others to share their thoughts and feelings by asking open-ended questions that invite keeper reflection and self-expression. Avoid leading or judgmental questions, and give them space to share their experiences at their own pace.

4. Practice Nonverbal Empathy: Pay attention to nonverbal cues such as facial expressions, body language, and tone of voice to better understand the emotions behind the words. Show empathy through your own nonverbal cues, such as nodding, making contact, and mirroring the person's body language.

5. Validate Their Feelings: Acknowledge and validate the other person's feelings, even if you don't agree with their perspective. Express empathy and understanding by saying things like, "I can see why you feel that way," or "It sounds like you're really struggling with this."

6. Cultivate Compassion: Cultivate a sense of compassion and kindness toward others, recognizing that everyone experiences pain, suffering, and challenges in life. Approach interactions with a genuine desire to alleviate suffering and promote well-being.

By developing empathy and understanding for others, you can strengthen your interpersonal relationships, enhance communication, and create a more compassionate and supportive social environment.

Developing emotional awareness is a journey of self-discovery and growth that requires practice, patience, and self-reflection. By recognizing and naming our own emotions, and building empathy and understanding for others, we can cultivate greater self-awareness, emotional intelligence, and interpersonal skills. As we deepen our emotional awareness, we become better equipped to navigate the complexities of human emotions and forge keeper, more meaningful connections with others.

Building and maintaining healthy relationships is essential for our emotional well-being and overall quality of life. Healthy relationships are characterized by mutual respect, trust, communication, and empathy. In this section, we'll explore two key aspects of building healthy relationships: conflict resolution skills and developing empathy and respect.

Conflict Resolution Skills

Conflict is a natural and inevitable part of any relationship, but how we handle conflicts can significantly impact the health and longevity of those relationships. Conflict resolution skills are essential for addressing disagreements, misunderstandings, and tensions in a constructive and respectful manner. Here are some strategies for developing effective conflict resolution skills:

1. Active Listening: Practice active listening by giving your full attention to the other person and focusing on understanding their perspective. Avoid interrupting or formulating your response while they're speaking. Instead, listen empathetically, paraphrase their points to ensure understanding, and ask clarifying questions if needed.

2. Expressing Yourself Assertively: Assertive communication involves expressing your thoughts, feelings, and needs clearly and respectfully, without resorting to aggression or passivity. Use "I" statements to express your feelings and avoid blaming or criticizing the other person. Be specific about the behavior or issue that is causing the conflict and focus on finding a mutually acceptable solution.

3. Finding Common Ground: Look for areas of agreement or common ground that can serve as a foundation for resolving the conflict. Focus on shared goals or interests and explore potential compromises or solutions that satisfy both parties' needs. Be open-minded and willing to consider alternative perspectives.

4. Managing Emotions: Keep your emotions in check during conflicts by practicing self-regulation techniques such as deep breathing, relaxation exercises, or taking a break if needed. Avoid escalating conflicts by resorting to personal attacks, yelling, or aggressive behavior. Instead, stay calm and focused on finding a resolution.

5. Seeking Mediation: If you're unable to resolve the conflict on your own, consider seeking the assistance of a neutral third party, such as a mediator or counselor. Mediators can facilitate constructive dialogue, help parties explorer underlying issues, and guide them toward mutually acceptable solutions.

6. Learning from Conflict: View conflict as an opportunity for growth and learning rather than as a sign of failure or inadequacy. Reflect on the underlying causes of the conflict, identify areas for improvement in communication or problem-solving, and commit to applying these lessons to future interactions.

By developing conflict resolution skills, you can effectively address conflicts when the rise, strengthen your relationships, and foster greater understanding and trust between you and others.

Developing Empathy and Respect
Empathy and respect are foundational elements of healthy relationships, allowing us to understand and appreciate the perspectives, feelings, and experiences of others. Developing empathy and respect involves cultivating a genuine concern for the well-being of others and treating them with dignity and kindness. Here's how to develop empathy and respect in your relationships:

1. Practice Active Listening: Actively listen to others without judgment or interruption, and strive to understand their feelings and perspectives. Put yourself in their shoes and imagine how you would feel in their situation. Show empathy by acknowledging their emotions and validating their experiences.

2. Show Genuine Interest: Demonstrate genuine interest in others by asking open-ended questions, showing curiosity about their lives and experiences, and actively engaging in conversation. Express empathy and concern for their well-being, and offer support and encouragement when needed.

3. Respect Boundaries: Respect the boundaries and personal space of others, both physical and emotional. Avoid intruding into areas that are private or sensitive without permission, and honor their right to set boundaries and assert their needs.

4. Practice Nonverbal Empathy: Pay attention to nonverbal cues such as facial expressions, body language, and tone of voice to better understand the emotions and intentions of others. Mirror their body language, make contact, and use attentive listening skills to convey empathy and respect.

5. Celebrate Diversity: Appreciate and calibrate the diversity of perspectives, backgrounds, and experiences that make each person unique. Embrace cultural differences, viewpoints, and identities, and strive to create an inclusive and accepting environment for everyone.

6. Show Kindness and Compassion: Demonstrate kindness and compassion toward others through your words and actions. Offer support, encouragement, and assistance when needed, and show appreciation for their contributions and efforts.

By developing empathy and respect in your relationships, you can foster deeper connections, build trust and mutual understanding, and create a positive and supportive social environment.

Building healthy relationships requires a combination of effective communication, conflict resolution skills, and empathy and respect. By developing essential skills and qualities, you can cultivate stronger, more meaningful relationships with others and create a supportive and nurturing social network. Remember that building healthy relationships is an ongoing process that requires effort, patience, and a commitment to mutual respect and understanding.

Coping with Anger in Challenging Situations

Anger is a natural response to challenging situations, but how we cope with anger can greatly impact our well-being and relationships. Learning to manage anger effectively in various contexts is essential for navigating the ups and downs of life. In this section, we'll explore strategies for coping with anger in challenging situations, including dealing with peer pressure, handling family conflict, and managing anger in academic and social settings.

Dealing with Peer Pressure

Peer pressure can trigger feelings of anger, frustration, and resentment, especially when it involves coercion or manipulation from peers. Learning to assert yourself and make decisions that align with your values and goals is key to coping with peer pressure effectively. Here are some strategies for dealing with peer pressure:

1. Know Your Values: Take time to reflect on your values, beliefs, and goals, and identify what is important to you. Having a clear sense of your values can help you make decisions that are consistent with your principles and priorities, even in the face of peer pressure.

2. Practice Assertiveness: Assertiveness involves standing up for yourself and expressing your thoughts, feelings, and needs in a confident and respectful manner. Practice saying "no" assertively when faced with peer pressure, and offer explanations or alternatives if necessary. Remember that it's okay to prioritize your own well-being and values over pleasing others.

3. Seek Support: Surround yourself with friends and peers who respect and support your choices, and seek out positive influences in your social circle. Having a support network of like-minded individuals can provide encouragement and validation when facing peer pressure.

4. Set Boundaries: Establish clear boundaries with your peers and communicate them assertively. Let others know what behaviors are acceptable to you and what are not, and be prepared to enforce your boundaries if they are crossed. Respect yourself enough to walk away from situations that compromise your values or integrity.

5. Practice Self-Care: Take care of yourself physically, emotionally, and mentally to build resilience to peer pressure. Engage in activities that bring you joy and fulfillment, prioritize your health and well-being, and practice self-compassion and self-acceptance.

By developing assertiveness skills, surrounding yourself with supportive peers, and prioritizing your own values and well-being, you can effectively cope with peer pressure and maintain healthy boundaries in your relationships.

Handling Family Conflict

Family conflict is a common source of anger and stress, but it's also an opportunity for growth, understanding, and reconciliation. Learning to communicate effectively, manage emotions, and find common ground can help you navigate family conflicts with greater ease. Here are some strategies for handling family conflict:

1. Practice Active Listening: Actively listen to the perspectives and concerns of family members without interrupting or becoming defensive. Show empathy and understanding, and strive to see the situation from their point of view. Reflect back what you hear to ensure understanding and validate their feelings.

2. Express Yourself Calmly: When expressing your own thoughts and feelings, do so calmly and respectfully. Avoid yelling, blaming, or criticizing others, as this can escalate conflicts and hinder effective communication. Use "I" statements to express your emotions and needs without placing blame.

3. Seek Common Ground: Look for areas of agreement or shared goals that can serve as a foundation for resolving the conflict. Focus on finding win-win solutions that address the needs and concerns of all family members involved. Be willing to compromise and negotiate in good faith.

4. Set Boundaries: Establish clear boundaries with family members and communicate them assertively. Let them know what behaviors are acceptable to you and what are not, and be prepared to enforce your boundaries if they are violated. Respect yourself enough to prioritize your own well-being and values.

5. Seek Mediation if Necessary: If conflicts persist and you're unable to resolve them on your own, consider seeking the assistance of a neutral third party, such as a family therapist or mediator. Mediators can facilitate constructive dialogue, help parties explorer underlying issues, and guide them toward mutually acceptable solutions.

By practicing active listening, expressing yourself calmly, seeking common ground, setting boundaries, and seeking mediation when needed, you can navigate family conflicts more effectively and strengthen your relationships with your loved ones.

Managing Anger in Academic and Social Settings

Academic and social settings can be breeding grounds for anger and frustration, especially when faced with academic pressure, peer conflicts, or social challenges. Learning to manage anger in these settings is essential for maintaining focus, resilience, and positive relationships. Here are some strategies for managing anger in academic and social settings:

1. Practice Stress Management: Develop healthy coping strategies for managing academic stress, such as time management, organization, and self-care. Take breaks when needed, prioritize tasks, and seek support from teachers, counselors, or academic advisors if you're feeling overwhelmed.

2. Communicate Effectively: When faced with conflicts or misunderstandings in academic or social settings, communicate your thoughts and feelings assertively and respectfully. Use "I" statements to express yourself and avoid blaming or attacking others. Listen actively to the perspectives of others and seek common ground.

3. Seek Support: Don't hesitate to seek support from teachers, peers, or mental health professionals if you're struggling with anger or stress in academic or social settings. They can offer guidance, resources, and strategies for coping with academic pressure, social challenges, and interpersonal conflicts.

4. Practice Self-Compassion: Be kind and compassionate toward yourself when facing challenges or setbacks in academic or social settings. Acknowledge your efforts and accomplishments, and remind yourself that it's okay to make mistakes or ask for help. Treat yourself with the understanding and empathy that you would offer to a friend.

5. Build Resilience: Cultivate resilient to academic and social stressors by focusing on your strengths, developing problem-solving skills, and maintaining a positive outlook. Embrace challenges as opportunities for growth and learning, and view setbacks as temporary obstacles rather than insurmountable barriers.

By practicing stress management, communicating effectively, seeking support, practicing self-compassion, and building resilience, you can effectively manage anger and navigate academic and social settings with greater ease and confidence.

Seeking Support

Seeking support is a crucial aspect of coping with anger and managing challenging situations effectively. Whether you're facing personal struggles, relationship conflicts, or academic stress, reaching out for support can provide guidance, validation, and resources to help you navigate through difficult times. In this section, we'll explore two important avenues for seeking support: identifying trusted adults and mentors, and accessing professional help and counseling options.

Identifying Trusted Adults and Mentors
Trusted adults and mentors play a vital role in providing guidance, encouragement, and support during challenging times. These individuals can offer a listening ear, practical advice, and emotional validation, helping you gain perspective and navigate through difficult situations. Here are some tips for identifying trusted adults and mentors in your life:

1. Family Members: Family members, such as parents, grandparents, or older siblings, can serve as trusted adults and mentors. They often have a deep understanding of your background, values, and personal history, making them valuable sources of support and guidance.

2. Teachers and School Counselors: Teachers and school counselors are trained professionals who can offer support and guidance in academic and personal matters. They can provide resources, referrals, and practical advice for coping with academic stress, peer conflicts, and other challenges.

3. Coaches and Extracurricular Leaders: Coaches, club advisors, and extracurricular leaders can serve as mentors and role models, offering guidance, encouragement, and support outside of the classroom. They may provide opportunities for skill-building, personal growth, and leadership development.

4. Community Leaders and Mentors: Community leaders, such as religious leaders, community organizers, or volunteer mentors, can offer valuable support and guidance in navigating community issues, cultural challenges, or personal struggles. They may provide mentorship, counseling, or referrals to community resources.

5. Healthcare Providers: Healthcare providers, such as doctors, therapists, or counselors, can offer support and guidance for physical, emotional, and mental health concerns. They can provide assessments, diagnoses, and treatment options for managing anger, stress, or other psychological issues.

When identifying trusted adults and mentors, look for individuals who demonstrate qualities such as empathy, respect, and trustworthiness. Consider their level of expertise, experience, and availability, and choose individuals who you feel comfortable confiding in and seeking guidance from.

Professional Help and Counseling Options

In addition to seeking support from trusted adults and mentors, professional help and counseling options can provide specialized assistance for managing anger, stress, and other psychological concerns. Professional counselors and therapists offer a safe and confidential space to explore your thoughts, feelings, and experiences, and can provide evidence-based interventions to help you cope and heal. Here are some professional help and counseling options to consider:

1. Individual Therapy: Individual therapy involves meeting one-on-one with a trained therapist or counselor to explore personal issues, set goals, and develop coping strategies for managing anger and other emotions. Therapists may use various therapeutic approaches, such as cognitive-behavioral therapy (CBT), dialectical behavior therapy (DBT), or mindfulness-based therapy, to address specific concerns and promote emotional well-being.

2. Group Therapy: Group therapy involves meeting with a small group of peers who share similar concerns or struggles, facilitated by a trained therapist or counselor. Group therapy provides opportunities for peer support, validation, and perspective-taking, and can be especially beneficial for learning new coping skills, practicing social interactions, and gaining insights from others' experiences.

3. Family Therapy: Family therapy involves meeting with a therapist or counselor as a family unit to address relationship conflicts, communication issues, and family dynamics. Family therapy provides a safe and supportive environment for exploring patterns of interaction, resolving conflicts, and strengthening family bonds.

4. Online Counseling: Online counseling platforms offer convenient and accessible options for receiving counseling and support from licensed therapists or counselors via phone, video, or text-based communication. Online counseling may be a suitable option for individuals who prefer the flexibility and privacy of virtual therapy sessions.

5. Psychiatric Evaluation and Medication Management: In some cases, anger and other psychological concerns may be related to underlying mental health conditions, such as depression, anxiety, or trauma. A psychiatric evaluation by a qualified psychiatrist or psychiatric nurse practitioner can provide diagnostic assessment, medication management, and treatment options tailored to your individual needs.

When considering professional help and counseling options, it's important to research and choose providers who are licensed, experienced, and knowledgeable in treating anger and related concerns. Consider factors such as cost, insurance coverage, location, and therapist qualifications, and don't hesitate to reach out for a consultation or initial assessment to determine if a provider is the right fit for you.

Seeking support from trusted adults, mentors, and professional counselors is an important aspect of coping with anger and managing challenging situations effectively. Whether you're facing personal struggles, relationship conflicts, or academic stress, reaching out for support can provide valuable guidance, validation, and resources to help you navigate through difficult times. Remember that seeking support is a sign of strength, not weakness, and that you don't have to face challenges alone. By reaching out for support and guidance, you can build resilience, gain perspective, and develop effective coping strategies for managing anger and promoting emotional well-being.

Moving Forward

As you work on managing anger and navigating through challenging situations, it's essential to focus on moving forward and taking proactive steps to promote personal growth and well-being. Setting goals for anger management and engaging in reflection and continuous improvement are key components of this process. In this section, we'll explore how setting goals and reflecting on your experiences can help you move forward on your journey toward healthier emotional expression and interpersonal relationships.

Setting Goals for Anger Management

Setting specific, measurable, achievable, relevant, and time-bound (SMART) goals for anger management can provide direction and motivation for your efforts to change and grow. These goals can range from short-term objectives to long-term aspirations, and they should be tailored to your individual needs, preferences, and circumstances. Here are some examples of SMART goals for anger management:

1. Short-Term Goal: "Practice deep breathing and relaxation exercises for 10 minutes each day to reduce stress and prevent anger from escalating."

2. Medium-Term Goal: "Attend a six-week anger management workshop to learn new coping strategies and communication skills for managing anger in challenging situations."

3. Long-Term Goal: "Develop healthy conflict resolution skills and maintain positive relationships with family members by attending family therapy sessions regularly and practicing open communication."

When setting goals for anger management, it's important to break them down into smaller, manageable steps and celebrate your progress along the way. Be flexible and adaptable in adjusting your goals as needed based on your evolving needs and circumstances, and don't be discouraged by setbacks or obstacles. Remember that change takes time and effort, and that every step forward is a step toward great emotional well-being and resilience.

Reflection and Continuous Improvement

Reflection is a powerful tool for self-awareness, learning, and growth. By taking time to reflect on your experiences, thoughts, and behaviors, you can gain insight into the underlying causes of your anger, identify patterns and triggers, and develop strategies for managing anger more effectively. Here are some strategies for reflection and continuous improvement:

1. Keep a Journal: Maintain a journal where you can record your thoughts, feelings, and experiences related to anger and its management. Use journaling as an opportunity for self-reflection, exploration, and problem-solving, and review your entries regularly to track your progress and identify areas for improvement.

2. Seek Feedback: Ask trusted friends, family members, or mentors for feedback on your anger management efforts. They may offer valuable insights, perspectives, and suggestions for coping with anger more effectively, and their support can provide encouragement and motivation for your journey.

3. Evaluate Your Strategies: Periodically evaluate the effectiveness of your anger management strategies and coping mechanisms. Assess what is working well and what could be improved, and be willing to experiment with new approaches and techniques based on your insights and feedback.

4. Celebrate Success: Celebrate your successes and accomplishments, no matter how small they may seem. Recognize and acknowledge your progress in managing anger and achieving your goals, and use victories as motivation to continue moving forward on your journey of personal growth and development.

5. Practice Self-Compassion: Be gentle and compassionate with yourself as you navigate the ups and downs of anger management. Accept that setbacks and challenges are a natural part of the process, and treat yourself with kindness, understanding, and patience as you work toward positive change.

By engaging in reflection and continuous improvement, you can deepen your self-awareness, refine your coping skills, and cultivate greater resilience in managing anger and related challenges. Embrace the process of growth and learning, and trust in your ability to overcome obstacles and thrive in the face of adversity.

Setting goals for anger management and engaging in reflection and continuous improvement are essential steps in moving forward on your journey toward healthier emotional expression and interpersonal relationships. By setting SMART goals, celebrating success, and learning from setbacks, you can chart a course toward greater self-awareness, emotional well-being, and resilience. Remember that change is a gradual process, and that every effort you make to manage anger more effectively brings you closer to living a life characterized by peace, balance, and fulfillment.

Conclusion

In conclusion, "Anger Management for Teen Boys" is not just a guide; it's a roadmap to empowerment, resilience, and growth. Throughout this journey, we explored the depths of anger, learned strategies for effective management, and embraced the importance of seeking support and continuous self-improvement.

From understanding the roots of anger to developing empathy, communication skills, and coping mechanisms, each chapter has been a stepping stone toward greater emotional intelligence and healthier relationships. We've navigated through challenging situations, acknowledging setbacks as opportunities for learning and growth.

As you close this book, remember that managing anger is not about suppressing emotions, but about harnessing their power constructively. It's about recognizing your triggers, embracing self-awareness, and choosing how to respond with intention and integrity.

You are not defined by your anger; you are defined by how you rise above it. Embrace the journey of self-discovery, celebrate your victories, and extend compassion to yourself along the way.

May this book serve as a beacon of hope and guidance as you navigate the complexities of adolescence and emerge stronger, wiser, and more resilient than ever before. The path forward may be challenging, but with courage, determination, and the tools you've gained, you have the power to create a future filled with peace, understanding, and boundless potential.

Remember: you are not alone, and your journey toward anger management is a testament to your strength, courage, and capacity for growth. Embrace the lessons learned, carry them forward, and step boldly into the bright future that awaits you.

www.ingramcontent.com/pod-product-compliance
Lightning Source LLC
Chambersburg PA
CBHW050839260726